The Complete Guide To Cardiovascular Disease

Understanding, Preventing, and treating Heart Disease

By

Dr. Gregory K. Edward

Copyright © by Dr. Gregory K. Edward 2022. All rights reserved. Before this document is duplicated or reproduced in any manner, the publisher's consent must be gained. Therefore, the contents within can neither be stored electronically, transferred, nor kept in a database. Neither in Part nor full can the document be copied, scanned, faxed, or retained without approval from the publisher or creator.

About The Author

Dr. Gregory Edward is a board-certified cardiologist and a Fellow of the American College of Cardiology. He has been practicing cardiology for over 25 years and has extensive experience in the diagnosis, treatment, and prevention of cardiovascular diseases. Dr. Edward received his medical degree from the University of Michigan Medical School and completed his residency in internal medicine at the University of Michigan Hospitals. He then completed a fellowship in cardiovascular disease at the University of Michigan Hospitals. Dr. Edward is a highly respected cardiologist and has been published in numerous medical journals, including the American Heart Journal, the Journal of the American College of Cardiology, and the New England Journal of Medicine. He is also a frequent speaker at national and international conferences on cardiovascular disease. Dr. Edward is passionate about helping patients understand and manage their cardiovascular health. He has written Cardiovascular Disease to provide readers with an in-depth look at the causes, diagnosis, and treatment of cardiovascular diseases. He hopes that his book will help readers make informed decisions about their health and take steps to reduce their risk of cardiovascular disease.

Table Of Contents

About The Author
Dear Friend,
Introduction to Cardiovascular Disease
Types of Cardiovascular Disease
Risk Factors for Cardiovascular Disease

Chapter 1
Heart Attacks
Causes of a Heart Attack
Treatment of a Heart Attack
Chapter 2
Stroke
Symptoms of a Stroke
Causes of a Stroke
Treatment of a Stroke

Chapter 3
Hypertension (High Blood Pressure)
Symptoms of High Blood Pressure
Treatment of High Blood Pressure
Chapter 4
Prevention and Management of
Cardiovascular Disease
Medical Treatment for Cardiovascular
Disease
Alternative Therapies for Cardiovascular
Disease
Conclusion
The Importance of Maintaining a Healthy
Cardiovascular System
Steps to Take for Cardiovascular Disease
Prevention and Management

Dear Friend,

Many individuals have recently been diagnosed with heart disease, and you may be one of them. Many others are in a similar predicament to you, so you are not alone. You don't have to accept your health as it is; you have the power to change. Heart disease results in real and significant misery. Don't assume that you will always have a heart ailment; taking care of it now will help you avoid problems later.

Heart disease is a common problem that 15% of the world's population faces. The heart, despite its small size, is vital to life; without it, people could not exist. The brain and other vital organs may get an ongoing supply of nutrients and oxygen thanks to the volume of blood the heart pumps. In addition to controlling blood pressure, it is responsible for pumping hormones and other significant molecules to different parts of the body, receiving deoxygenated blood and moving metabolic waste products from the body to the lungs for oxygenation. This vital organ may be harmed in a variety of ways. Important risk factors for cardiovascular disease include hypertension, high cholesterol, obesity, smoking, diabetes, inactivity, and heredity. Atherosclerotic plaque formation in the arteries restricts blood flow from the heart.

Introduction to Cardiovascular Disease

It was a typical Saturday morning for 45-year-old Jack. He woke up early, as he always did, and headed to his favorite coffee shop for his daily caffeine fix. As he walked to the shop, he felt a sudden, sharp pain in his chest. He collapsed to the ground, clutching his chest and gasping for air.

A passerby saw Jack lying on the ground and immediately called 911. Within minutes, an ambulance arrived and rushed Jack to the hospital. At the hospital, the doctors determined that Jack was experiencing a heart attack.

They quickly performed emergency surgery to clear the blockage in Jack's coronary artery and restore blood flow to his heart.

After the surgery, Jack was told that he had a history of high cholesterol and high blood pressure, both of which put him at higher risk for a heart attack. He had never paid much attention to his cardiovascular health, and it had caught up with him.

The experience was a wake-up call for Jack. He realized the importance of taking care of his cardiovascular system and made lifestyle changes to improve his health. He started eating a healthier diet, exercising regularly, and taking his medications as prescribed.

Thanks to the timely intervention of the ambulance and the skilled care of the hospital staff, Jack made a full recovery. He learned a valuable lesson about the importance of taking care of his heart and vowed to prioritize his cardiovascular health for the rest of his life.

Cardiovascular disease, also known as heart disease, is a term used to describe a range of conditions that affect the heart and blood vessels. These conditions can include coronary artery disease, heart attacks, heart failure, and stroke, among others. Cardiovascular disease is a leading cause of death and disability worldwide, and it can affect people of all ages and backgrounds.

There are several risk factors for cardiovascular disease, including high blood pressure, high cholesterol, smoking, diabetes, and a family history of cardiovascular disease. Many of these risk factors can be controlled or modified through lifestyle changes, such as eating a healthy diet, exercising regularly, and not smoking.

Early detection and treatment of cardiovascular disease is important in order to prevent or manage the condition and reduce the risk of serious complications. This may involve a combination of lifestyle changes, medical treatment, and alternative therapies, depending on the individual case. By taking steps to maintain a healthy cardiovascular system, we can greatly reduce the risk of developing cardiovascular disease and improve our overall health and well-being.

Definition of Cardiovascular Disease
Cardiovascular disease, also known as heart disease, is a term used to describe a range of conditions that affect the heart and blood vessels. These conditions can include coronary artery disease, heart attacks, heart failure, and stroke, among others. Cardiovascular disease is a leading cause of death and disability worldwide, and it can affect people of all ages and backgrounds.

Cardiovascular disease is characterized by problems with the function and structure of the heart and blood vessels.

These problems can occur as a result of a variety of factors, including genetics, lifestyle choices, and underlying health conditions. Some common forms of cardiovascular disease include:

Coronary artery disease: This occurs when the arteries that supply blood to the heart become narrowed or blocked, often due to the build-up of plaque. This can lead to chest pain (angina) and, in severe cases, a heart attack.

Heart failure: This occurs when the heart is unable to pump enough blood to meet the body's needs. It can be caused by a variety of factors, including high blood pressure, coronary artery disease, and heart attacks.

Stroke: This occurs when a blood clot blocks the flow of blood to the brain, or when a blood vessel in the brain ruptures. This can lead to brain damage and other serious complications.

Cardiovascular disease can have serious consequences if left untreated, including heart attacks, heart failure, and stroke. It is important to be aware of the risk factors for cardiovascular disease and to take steps to prevent or manage the condition in order to maintain good heart health.

Types of Cardiovascular Disease

There are several types of cardiovascular disease, which can affect the heart and blood vessels in different ways. Some common types of cardiovascular disease include:

Coronary artery disease: This occurs when the arteries that supply blood to the heart become narrowed or blocked, often due to the build-up of plaque. This can lead to chest pain (angina) and, in severe cases, a heart attack.

Heart failure: This occurs when the heart is unable to pump enough blood to meet the body's needs. It can be caused by a variety of factors, including high blood pressure, coronary artery disease, and heart attacks.

Heart valve problems: The heart has four valves that control the flow of blood through the heart. When these valves become damaged or diseased, they may not function properly, leading to problems such as shortness of breath and fatigue.

Cardiomyopathy: This is a group of conditions that affect the heart muscle, making it harder for the heart to pump blood effectively. Cardiomyopathy can be caused by a variety of factors, including genetics, infections, and certain medications.

Aortic aneurysm: This occurs when the aorta, the main artery that carries blood away from the heart, becomes weakened and expands or bulges. This can be a serious condition if the aneurysm ruptures.

Stroke: This occurs when a blood clot blocks the flow of blood to the brain, or when a blood vessel in the brain ruptures. This can lead to brain damage and other serious complications.

It is important to be aware of the different types of cardiovascular disease and to understand the signs and symptoms of each condition. Early detection and treatment can help prevent or manage cardiovascular disease and reduce the risk of serious complications.

Risk Factors for Cardiovascular Disease

There are several risk factors for cardiovascular disease, which is a term used to describe a range of conditions that affect the heart and blood vessels. These conditions can include coronary artery disease, heart attacks, heart failure, and stroke, among others. Some common risk factors for cardiovascular disease include:

High blood pressure: High blood pressure, or hypertension, puts extra strain on the heart and blood vessels, increasing the risk of cardiovascular disease.

High cholesterol: High levels of cholesterol in the blood can increase the risk of plaque build-up in the arteries, which can lead to coronary artery disease and heart attacks.

Smoking: Smoking damages the blood vessels and increases the risk of plaque build-up in the arteries, as well as increasing the risk of lung cancer and other respiratory problems.

Diabetes: People with diabetes are at increased risk of cardiovascular disease, as high blood sugar levels can damage the blood vessels and increase the risk of plaque build-up.

Age: Cardiovascular disease is more common in older adults, although it can affect people of all ages.

Family history: If you have a family history of cardiovascular disease, you may be at an increased risk of developing the condition yourself.

Lack of physical activity: A sedentary lifestyle can increase the risk of cardiovascular disease, as regular exercise can help keep the heart and blood vessels healthy.

Poor diet: A diet high in saturated and trans fats, salt, and processed foods can increase the risk of cardiovascular disease.

Understanding and addressing these risk factors can help prevent or manage cardiovascular disease and reduce the risk of serious complications.

Chapter 1

Heart Attacks

It was a typical Wednesday morning when Maria's life changed forever. She had just dropped her kids off at school and was getting ready to start her day when she suddenly felt a crushing pain in her chest. She tried to ignore it, thinking it was just a muscle spasm, but the pain only got worse. She began to feel lightheaded and short of breath, and she knew something was seriously wrong.

She called out for her husband, who was in the next room, and told him she thought she was having a heart attack. He called 911 and helped her lay down on the couch, trying to stay calm as they waited for the ambulance to arrive. Maria was terrified, not just because of the pain she was in, but because she had always been careful about her health. She exercised regularly, ate a healthy diet, and didn't smoke. She couldn't understand how this could be happening to her.

The ambulance arrived quickly and the paramedics rushed her to the hospital, where she was immediately seen by a team of doctors and nurses. They told her she had indeed had a heart attack and needed to have a procedure to open up the blocked artery in her heart. Maria was terrified, but she knew she had no choice. She trusted her doctors and knew they would do everything they could to save her.

The procedure was a success, and Maria spent the next few days in the hospital recovering. It was a scary and difficult experience, but she was grateful to be alive. She knew she had to make some changes to her lifestyle in order to prevent another heart attack from happening, and she was determined to do everything she could to stay healthy.

Maria's heart attack was a wake-up call, and it made her realize just how fragile and precious life can be. She was grateful to have received timely and effective treatment, and she knew that she needed to take better care of herself in order to prevent another heart attack from happening. She made a commitment to live a healthier lifestyle and to prioritize her health, and she knew that she could overcome this challenge and come out stronger on the other side.

A heart attack, also known as a myocardial infarction, is a serious medical emergency that occurs when the blood flow to the heart is blocked, causing damage to the heart muscle. This can be caused by a blockage in one or more of the coronary arteries, which supply blood to the heart. Heart attacks are a leading cause of death and disability worldwide, and they can occur at any age.

Symptoms of a heart attack can include chest pain or discomfort, shortness of breath, nausea, vomiting, and pain in the arms, neck, jaw, or back. If someone is experiencing these symptoms, it is important to call emergency services immediately. Heart attacks require immediate medical attention in order to prevent serious damage to the heart muscle.

There are several risk factors for heart attacks, including high blood pressure, high cholesterol, smoking, diabetes, and a family history of heart disease. Many of these risk factors can be controlled or modified through lifestyle changes, such as eating a healthy diet, exercising regularly, and not smoking.

Treatment for a heart attack typically involves medications to restore blood flow to the heart, as well as procedures to remove the blockage from the artery. In severe cases, surgery may be necessary to repair or bypass the blocked artery. After a heart attack, it is important to follow the recommended treatment plan in order to prevent future heart attacks and manage any underlying health conditions.

Symptoms of a Heart Attack
The symptoms of a heart attack can vary from person to person, and not everyone will experience all of the following symptoms:

Chest pain or discomfort: This is the most common symptom of a heart attack, and it can feel like a crushing or squeezing sensation in the chest. The pain may also spread to the arms, neck, jaw, or back.

Shortness of breath: A person experiencing a heart attack may feel short of breath, even when they are not physically active.

Nausea and vomiting: Some people may feel sick to their stomach or vomit during a heart attack.

Sweating: A person experiencing a heart attack may break out in a cold sweat.

Lightheadedness or fainting: A person may feel lightheaded or faint during a heart attack.

It is important to be aware of the symptoms of a heart attack and to seek medical attention immediately if you or someone else is experiencing these symptoms. Timely treatment can help prevent serious damage to the heart muscle and increase the chances of survival.

Causes of a Heart Attack

It was a hot summer day, and all Sarah wanted to do was relax by the pool with a cold drink and a good book. She had been working hard all year and deserved a break, and she was looking forward to spending a few days at her family's summer home by the beach.

As she settled into her lounge chair, she noticed that her heart was beating faster than usual. She chalked it up to the heat and the excitement of being on vacation, and she tried to focus on her book. But the racing of her heart only seemed to get worse, and she began to feel lightheaded and short of breath.

She sat up and tried to take deep breaths, but nothing seemed to help. She called out for her husband, who was lounging nearby, and told him she thought something was wrong. He immediately sprang into action, calling 911 and helping her lay down on the ground.

Sarah was terrified, not just because of the physical symptoms she was experiencing, but because she had always been careful about her health. She exercised regularly, ate a healthy diet, and didn't smoke. She couldn't understand how this could be happening to her.

The ambulance arrived quickly and the paramedics rushed her to the hospital, where she was immediately seen by a team of doctors and nurses. They told her she had had a heart attack and needed to have a procedure to open up the blocked artery in her heart. Sarah was terrified, but she knew she had no choice. She trusted her doctors and knew they would do everything they could to save her.

The procedure was a success, and Sarah spent the next few days in the hospital recovering. It was a scary and difficult experience, but she was grateful to be alive. She knew she had to make some changes to her lifestyle in order to prevent another heart attack from happening, and she was determined to do everything she could to stay healthy.

Sarah's heart attack was a wake-up call, and it made her realize just how fragile and precious life can be. She was grateful to have received timely and effective treatment, and she knew that she needed to take better care of herself in order to prevent another heart attack from happening. She made a commitment to live a healthier lifestyle and to prioritize her health, and she knew that she could overcome this challenge and come out stronger on the other side.

A heart attack, also known as a myocardial infarction, is a serious medical emergency that occurs when the blood flow to the heart is blocked, causing damage to the heart muscle. There are several factors that can increase the risk of a heart attack, including:

Coronary artery disease: This is the most common cause of heart attacks, and it occurs when the arteries that supply blood to the heart become narrowed or blocked, often due to the build-up of plaque. Plaque is a sticky substance made up of fat, cholesterol, and other substances in the blood. When plaque builds up in the arteries, it can reduce or block the flow of blood to the heart, leading to a heart attack.

Blood clots: A blood clot can form in one of the coronary arteries and block the flow of blood to the heart, leading to a heart attack. Blood clots can be caused by a variety of factors, including high blood pressure, high cholesterol, and smoking.

Physical stress: Physical stress, such as extreme physical exertion or emotional stress, can increase the risk of a heart attack.

Other factors: Other factors that can increase the risk of a heart attack include high blood pressure, high cholesterol, diabetes, obesity, and a family history of heart disease.

It is important to be aware of the risk factors for heart attacks and to take steps to reduce these risks in order to prevent a heart attack from occurring. This may involve lifestyle changes, such as eating a healthy diet, exercising regularly, and not smoking, as well as taking medications as prescribed to manage underlying health conditions.

Treatment of a Heart Attack

It is important to note that the primary treatment for a heart attack is seeking emergency medical care. Medications and procedures, such as coronary angioplasty or coronary artery bypass surgery, may be necessary to restore blood flow to the heart and prevent further damage to the heart muscle.

That being said, there are some natural remedies that may be helpful in managing the symptoms of a heart attack and supporting overall heart health. These remedies should not be used as a substitute for medical treatment, but rather as a complementary approach to care. Some natural remedies for heart attack may include:

Garlic: Garlic has been shown to have anti-inflammatory and cholesterol-lowering effects, which may help reduce the risk of heart attacks.

Ginger: Ginger has been shown to have anti-inflammatory and blood-thinning effects, which may help reduce the risk of heart attacks.

Turmeric: Turmeric has been shown to have anti-inflammatory and cholesterol-lowering effects, which may help reduce the risk of heart attacks.

Coenzyme Q10: Coenzyme Q10 is an antioxidant that is found in the body and is thought to have a protective effect on the heart.

Omega-3 fatty acids: Omega-3 fatty acids, which are found in fatty fish like salmon and mackerel, have been shown to have a protective effect on the heart.

It is important to speak with a healthcare provider before starting any new natural remedies, as some may interact with medications or have potential side effects. It is also important to follow the recommended treatment plan for a heart attack in order to prevent further damage to the heart muscle and manage any underlying health conditions.

Dr. Edward's brother, David, had always been careful about his health. He ate a healthy diet, exercised regularly, and didn't smoke. So when he started experiencing chest pain one evening, he didn't think much of it. He figured it was just indigestion or a muscle spasm.

But as the pain persisted and grew worse, David began to worry. He called his brother, Dr. Edward, who was a cardiologist, and explained his symptoms. Dr. Edward told him to call 911 immediately and go to the hospital.
He knew that heart attacks could sometimes present with mild symptoms, and he didn't want to take any chances.

David arrived at the hospital and was seen by a team of doctors and nurses.

They confirmed that he was indeed having a heart attack and quickly began treatment to restore blood flow to his heart. They gave him medications to break up the blood clot in his artery and prepared him for a procedure to remove the blockage.

Dr. Edward stayed by his brother's side throughout the entire process, offering support and encouragement. He knew that heart attacks could be a scary and overwhelming experience, and he wanted to be there for his brother every step of the way.

After the procedure, David was taken to the intensive care unit to recover. He was hooked up to monitors and given medications to help his heart heal. Dr.

Edward stayed with him, keeping a close eye on his progress.

As David recovered, Dr. Edward made a point to talk to him about natural treatment options for heart health. He knew that there were many lifestyle changes and alternative therapies that could help prevent future heart attacks and support heart health. He encouraged his brother to adopt a healthy diet, exercise regularly, and try stress-reducing techniques like meditation and yoga.

David was grateful for his brother's guidance and support. He knew that he had a long road to recovery ahead of him, but he was determined to take control of his health and do everything he could to prevent another heart attack from happening. With his brother's help and support, he was confident that he could overcome this challenge and live a healthy, heart-healthy life.

A heart attack, also known as a myocardial infarction, is a serious medical emergency that occurs when the blood flow to the heart is blocked, causing damage to the heart muscle. If someone is experiencing a heart attack, it is important to call emergency services immediately, as prompt treatment is essential to prevent serious damage to the heart muscle.

The main goal of treatment for a heart attack is to restore blood flow to the heart as quickly as possible. This may involve a combination of medications and procedures, such as:

Medications: Medications can be used to break up blood clots and restore blood flow to the heart. These may include aspirin, blood thinners, and other medications.

Coronary artery angioplasty and stenting: This is a procedure in which a balloon catheter is inserted into the blocked artery and inflated to open up the blockage. A stent, which is a small mesh tube, may also be inserted to help keep the artery open.

Coronary artery bypass surgery: This is a more complex procedure in which a healthy blood vessel from another part of the body is used to bypass the blocked artery and restore blood flow to the heart.

After a heart attack, it is important to follow the recommended treatment plan in order to prevent future heart attacks and manage any underlying health conditions. This may involve lifestyle changes, such as eating a healthy diet, exercising regularly, and not smoking, as well as taking medications as prescribed. It is also important to follow up with a healthcare provider regularly to monitor progress and make any necessary adjustments to the treatment plan.

Chapter 2

Stroke

It was a typical Wednesday afternoon when Jane received the devastating news. Her husband, Tom, had suffered a massive stroke while at work. She could hardly believe it as she rushed to the hospital, her mind racing with fear and uncertainty.

When she arrived at the hospital, she was met with the grim reality of Tom's condition. He was unconscious, with tubes and wires connecting him to various machines. The doctors and nurses were working frantically to stabilize him, but Jane could see the worry on their faces.

As the days passed, Jane kept a constant vigil at Tom's bedside, praying for his recovery. She watched as he struggled to communicate, his once-strong body now weak and fragile. It was a heart-wrenching sight, and Jane couldn't help but feel helpless and overwhelmed.

But despite the challenges, Tom was determined to fight. He worked tirelessly with physical therapists and speech therapists, determined to regain his strength and independence. And slowly but surely, he began to make progress.

As the weeks turned into months, Tom's recovery became more and more miraculous. He was able to speak again, and even walk with the help of a cane. And though he would always carry the scars of his stroke, he was grateful to be alive and to have his wife by his side.

For Jane, the journey had been filled with tears and heartache, but also with love and hope. And as she watched Tom walk out of the hospital, a new sense of determination and resilience in his step, she knew that they had overcome one of the toughest challenges of their lives.

A stroke is a serious and life-threatening medical condition that occurs when the blood supply to the brain is disrupted. This can be due to a blockage in the blood vessels, known as an ischemic stroke, or a rupture of a blood vessel, known as a hemorrhagic stroke. Either way, the lack of oxygen-rich blood to the brain can cause damage to brain cells and lead to serious problems.

Symptoms of a stroke may include sudden numbness or weakness in the face, arm, or leg, especially on one side of the body; difficulty speaking or understanding speech; trouble seeing in one or both eyes; difficulty walking, dizziness, or loss of balance and coordination; and severe headache with no known cause. These symptoms often occur suddenly and may progress quickly.

If you or someone you know is experiencing these symptoms, it is important to seek medical attention immediately. Time is of the essence when it comes to treating a stroke, as the longer the brain is deprived of oxygen, the more severe the damage can be.

Treatment for a stroke may include medications to dissolve blood clots or stop bleeding, surgery to repair damaged blood vessels, and rehabilitation to help the patient regain their abilities. The type of treatment will depend on the type and severity of the stroke.

Preventing a stroke involves making lifestyle changes, such as quitting smoking, maintaining a healthy diet, and exercising regularly. It is also important to manage any underlying health conditions, such as high blood pressure, diabetes, and heart disease, as these can increase the risk of stroke.

Strokes can have serious and long-lasting effects, including paralysis, difficulty speaking or swallowing, memory loss, and difficulty with daily activities. However, with prompt medical attention and proper treatment and rehabilitation, many people are able to make a full or partial recovery from a stroke.

Symptoms of a Stroke

The symptoms of a stroke can vary depending on the severity of the condition and the area of the brain that is affected. Some common symptoms of a stroke include:

1. Sudden numbness or weakness in the face, arm, or leg, especially on one side of the body
2. Difficulty speaking or understanding speech
3. Trouble seeing in one or both eyes
4. Difficulty walking, dizziness, or loss of balance and coordination
5. Severe headache with no known cause

It is important to note that these symptoms often occur suddenly and may progress quickly. If you or someone you know is experiencing any of these symptoms, it is crucial to seek medical attention immediately. Time is of the essence when it comes to treating a stroke, as the longer the brain is deprived of oxygen, the more severe the damage can be. Other symptoms of a stroke may include difficulty swallowing, changes in mood or behavior, and changes in sensory abilities.

Causes of a Stroke

A stroke is caused by a disruption in the blood supply to the brain, which can occur in two ways: an ischemic stroke or a hemorrhagic stroke.

An ischemic stroke is the most common type of stroke and occurs when a blood vessel in the brain becomes blocked, usually by a blood clot. This prevents oxygen-rich blood from reaching the brain, which can cause damage to brain cells.

A hemorrhagic stroke is less common, but more serious, and occurs when a blood vessel in the brain ruptures and bleeds into the surrounding tissue. This can cause damage to brain cells and disrupt the normal functioning of the brain.

There are several risk factors that can increase the likelihood of having a stroke, including:

1. High blood pressure: High blood pressure puts extra strain on the

blood vessels, which can lead to a stroke.
2. Smoking: Smoking damages the blood vessels and increases the risk of blood clots, which can lead to a stroke.
3. Diabetes: High blood sugar levels can damage blood vessels and increase the risk of a stroke.
4. High cholesterol: High cholesterol levels can build up in the blood vessels and increase the risk of a stroke.
5. Heart disease: Heart conditions such as atrial fibrillation, heart attack, and heart failure can increase the risk of a stroke.
6. Age: The risk of having a stroke increases as we get older.

7. Family history: Having a family member who has had a stroke increases the risk of having a stroke.
8. Gender: Men are more likely to have a stroke than women.
9. Ethnicity: Some ethnic groups, such as African Americans and Hispanics, have a higher risk of stroke.

It is important to manage these risk factors to reduce the likelihood of having a stroke. This may involve making lifestyle changes, such as quitting smoking and maintaining a healthy diet, and managing any underlying health conditions, such as high blood pressure and diabetes.

Treatment of a Stroke

Janine had always been an active and healthy person, but one day, she suddenly experienced weakness on one side of her body and difficulty speaking.

She immediately knew something was wrong and called for an ambulance.

At the hospital, the doctors determined that Janine had suffered a stroke and needed immediate treatment. They administered a medication called tPA, which helps to dissolve blood clots and improve blood flow to the brain. They also performed a CT scan to determine the extent of the stroke and the best course of treatment.

The results of the CT scan showed that Janine had an ischemic stroke, caused by a blood clot in one of the blood vessels in her brain. The doctors decided to perform a procedure called an endovascular clot removal, which involves threading a small catheter through the blood vessels to the site of the clot and removing it.

The procedure was a success and Janine began to show improvement almost immediately. However, she still faced a long road to recovery. She received physical, occupational, and speech therapy to help her regain her abilities and independence. She also had to make lifestyle changes, such as quitting smoking and eating a healthier diet, to reduce her risk of having another stroke.

After several months of hard work, Janine was able to return to her normal activities and was grateful for the timely treatment that had saved her life. She knew that if she had not sought medical attention right away, the outcome could have been much different. She made it her mission to educate others about the importance of recognizing the symptoms of a stroke and seeking treatment immediately.

The treatment of a stroke depends on the type and severity of the condition. The most common treatments for a stroke include:

Medications: Medications such as tPA (tissue plasminogen activator) can be used to dissolve blood clots and improve blood flow to the brain in cases of an ischemic stroke. Anticoagulants may also be used to prevent blood clots from forming. For a hemorrhagic stroke, medications may be used to stop the bleeding and lower blood pressure.

Surgery: In some cases, surgery may be needed to repair damaged blood vessels or remove blood clots. This may include procedures such as endovascular clot removal, carotid endarterectomy, or aneurysm repair.

Rehabilitation: Rehabilitation is an important part of the treatment process for a stroke. Physical, occupational, and speech therapy can help the patient regain their abilities and independence.

It is important to seek medical attention as soon as possible after experiencing the symptoms of a stroke, as time is of the essence in treating this condition. The longer the brain is deprived of oxygen, the more severe the damage can be.

In addition to medical treatment, making lifestyle changes, such as quitting smoking and maintaining a healthy diet, can help reduce the risk of having another stroke. It is also important to manage any underlying health conditions, such as high blood pressure and diabetes, to prevent future strokes.

While traditional medical treatment is crucial for managing a stroke, there are also natural treatments that may be helpful in the recovery process. These treatments may include:

Acupuncture: Acupuncture is a form of traditional Chinese medicine that involves the insertion of thin needles into specific points on the body to stimulate healing and improve circulation. It may be helpful in reducing the severity of stroke symptoms and improving overall recovery.

Massage therapy: Massage therapy can help to relax the muscles, improve circulation, and reduce stress, which may be beneficial for those recovering from a stroke.

Exercise: Regular exercise, such as walking, biking, or swimming, can help to improve mobility and strength, and may also have a positive effect on mood and overall well-being.

Diet: A healthy diet, rich in fruits, vegetables, and whole grains, can help to improve overall health and reduce the risk of stroke. Some studies have also shown that certain foods, such as fish, nuts, and berries, may be particularly beneficial for stroke recovery.

Herbal remedies: Some herbs, such as ginkgo biloba and turmeric, have been shown to have a positive effect on brain function and may be helpful in the recovery process. However, it is important to speak with a healthcare provider before taking any herbal remedies, as they may interact with medications or have potential side effects.

It is important to note that natural treatments should not be used as a replacement for traditional medical treatment, but rather as a complement to it. It is always best to speak with a healthcare provider before starting any natural treatment regimen.

Chapter 3

Hypertension (High Blood Pressure)

Jackson had always been a bit of a stress-loving, Type A personality. He enjoyed the thrill of juggling multiple projects at work and pushing himself to the limit. However, one day, he began to notice that his chest felt tight and he was constantly feeling dizzy and lightheaded. He decided to visit his doctor, who checked his blood pressure and gave him some shocking news.

Jackson's blood pressure was through the roof and he was diagnosed with hypertension, or high blood pressure. His doctor explained that high blood pressure puts extra strain on the blood vessels, which can lead to serious health problems, such as heart attack, stroke, and kidney disease.

Jackson was shocked and realized that he needed to make some changes in his life to lower his blood pressure. He began taking blood pressure medications as prescribed by his doctor and made some lifestyle changes, such as quitting smoking, eating a healthier diet, and exercising regularly. He also learned relaxation techniques, such as meditation and deep breathing, to help manage stress.

It took some time and effort, but Jackson's blood pressure eventually came down to a healthy level. He was grateful that he had caught his condition early and made the necessary changes, as it had likely saved him from experiencing more serious health problems in the future. He learned to embrace a more balanced and healthy lifestyle, and his stress levels greatly improved as a result.

Hypertension, or high blood pressure, is a common medical condition that occurs when the force of the blood against the artery walls is too high. This puts extra strain on the blood vessels, which can lead to serious health problems, such as heart attack, stroke, and kidney disease.

High blood pressure is often referred to as the "silent killer" because it often has no noticeable symptoms. This is why it is important to have regular blood pressure check-ups, as it can be easily managed with lifestyle changes and medication if caught early.

Risk factors for high blood pressure include smoking, obesity, high salt intake, stress, and family history. It is also more common in older adults and those with certain medical conditions, such as diabetes and kidney disease.

To manage high blood pressure, it is important to make lifestyle changes, such as quitting smoking, eating a healthy diet, and exercising regularly. Medications may also be prescribed to help lower blood pressure. It is important to take medications as directed and continue with lifestyle changes to keep blood pressure at a healthy level.

If left untreated, high blood pressure can lead to serious health complications. However, with proper management, it is possible to live a healthy and active life with high blood pressure.

Symptoms of High Blood Pressure

High blood pressure, or hypertension, is often referred to as the "silent killer" because it often has no noticeable symptoms. However, in some cases, there may be some warning signs of high blood pressure, such as:

Headaches: People with high blood pressure may experience frequent or severe headaches, especially at the front of the head.

Chest pain: High blood pressure can cause chest pain or discomfort, especially during physical activity.

Shortness of breath: High blood pressure can make it difficult to catch your breath, even when you are resting.

Dizziness or lightheadedness: High blood pressure can cause dizziness or lightheadedness, especially when standing up quickly.

Nosebleeds: High blood pressure can cause the blood vessels in the nose to become more fragile, leading to frequent nosebleeds.

Flushing: Some people with high blood pressure may experience flushing, or a feeling of warmth in the face, neck, and chest.

If you are experiencing any of these symptoms, it is important to speak with a healthcare provider. High blood pressure can often be managed with lifestyle changes and medication if caught early. It is important to have regular blood pressure check-ups to ensure that it is kept at a healthy level.

Causes of High Blood Pressure

High blood pressure, or hypertension, is a common medical condition that occurs when the force of the blood against the artery walls is too high. This puts extra strain on the blood vessels, which can lead to serious health problems, such as heart attack, stroke, and kidney disease.

There are several factors that can contribute to the development of high blood pressure, including:

Age: High blood pressure is more common in older adults, especially those over the age of 60.

Genetics: A family history of high blood pressure increases the risk of developing the condition.

Lifestyle factors: Smoking, obesity, high salt intake, and lack of physical activity can all increase the risk of high blood pressure.

Medical conditions: Certain medical conditions, such as diabetes, kidney disease, and sleep apnea, can increase the risk of high blood pressure.

Stress: Chronic stress can lead to high blood pressure.

It is important to manage these risk factors to reduce the likelihood of developing high blood pressure. This may involve making lifestyle changes, such as quitting smoking and maintaining a healthy diet, and managing any underlying health conditions. It is also important to have regular blood pressure check-ups to ensure that it is kept at a healthy level.

Treatment of High Blood Pressure

High blood pressure, also known as hypertension, is a common condition that occurs when the force of blood against the artery walls is too high. If left untreated, it can lead to serious health problems such as heart disease, stroke, and kidney failure. While medication is often prescribed to manage high blood pressure, there are also natural ways to lower blood pressure and improve overall health.

One of the most effective natural treatments for high blood pressure is lifestyle modification. This includes eating a healthy diet that is low in salt and saturated fats, exercising regularly, and reducing stress. A diet rich in fruits, vegetables, and whole grains can help lower blood pressure, while processed foods and fast food should be avoided. Exercise, such as walking, running, or biking, can also help lower blood pressure and improve overall health.

Another natural treatment for high blood pressure is herbal remedies. Some herbs, such as garlic, ginger, and hawthorn, have been shown to have blood pressure-lowering effects. These herbs can be taken in supplement form or added to foods for flavor.

Another option for natural treatment of high blood pressure is relaxation techniques, such as meditation, yoga, or deep breathing. These practices can help reduce stress and lower blood pressure.

It is important to note that while natural treatments can be effective in managing high blood pressure, they should not be used as a replacement for medication prescribed by a healthcare professional. It is important to work with a healthcare provider to determine the best treatment plan for high blood pressure.

Treatment of high blood pressure, or hypertension, is essential to prevent serious health problems such as heart disease, stroke, and kidney failure. There are several ways to treat high blood pressure, including lifestyle modification, medication, and natural remedies.

Lifestyle modification is a key part of treating high blood pressure. This includes eating a healthy diet that is low in salt and saturated fats, exercising regularly, and reducing stress. A diet rich in fruits, vegetables, and whole grains can help lower blood pressure, while processed foods and fast food should be avoided. Exercise, such as walking, running, or biking, can also help lower blood pressure and improve overall health.

Medication is often prescribed to lower blood pressure and manage hypertension. Common types of blood pressure medications include diuretics, beta blockers, ACE inhibitors, and calcium channel blockers. These medications work by lowering blood pressure and reducing the risk of heart disease and stroke.

Natural remedies, such as herbal remedies and relaxation techniques, can also be used to treat high blood pressure. Herbs such as garlic, ginger, and hawthorn have been shown to have blood pressure-lowering effects and can be taken in supplement form or added to foods for flavor. Relaxation techniques, such as meditation, yoga, and deep breathing, can help reduce stress and lower blood pressure.

It is important to work with a healthcare provider to determine the best treatment plan for high blood pressure. This may involve a combination of lifestyle modification, medication, and natural remedies. It is also important to regularly monitor blood pressure levels and make any necessary adjustments to treatment.

Chapter 4

Prevention and Management of Cardiovascular Disease

Cardiovascular disease (CVD) refers to a group of conditions that affect the heart and blood vessels, including coronary artery disease, heart failure, stroke, and hypertension. CVD is a leading cause of death and disability worldwide, but it is also preventable and manageable through lifestyle changes, medication, and medical procedures.

Prevention of CVD begins with addressing risk factors that increase the likelihood of developing the disease. These risk factors include:

High blood pressure: Elevated blood pressure puts extra strain on the heart and blood vessels, increasing the risk of CVD.

High cholesterol: High levels of LDL cholesterol (the "bad" cholesterol) can contribute to the development of plaque in the arteries, increasing the risk of CVD.

Diabetes: People with diabetes have an increased risk of CVD because high blood sugar levels can damage blood vessels and the nerves that control the heart.

Obesity: Excess weight, especially abdominal fat, increases the risk of CVD.

Smoking: Smoking damages the blood vessels and increases the risk of CVD.

Lack of physical activity: Regular physical activity can help lower the risk of CVD by maintaining a healthy weight, controlling blood pressure, and improving cholesterol levels.

Poor diet: A diet high in saturated and trans fats, salt, and added sugars can increase the risk of CVD.

To prevent CVD, it is important to adopt a healthy lifestyle that includes:

Eating a healthy diet that is rich in fruits, vegetables, whole grains, and lean proteins.

Getting regular physical activity, such as at least 150 minutes of moderate-intensity exercise per week.

Not smoking or using tobacco products.

Maintaining a healthy weight.

Managing stress through techniques such as meditation, yoga, or deep breathing.

Getting regular check-ups and screenings to monitor blood pressure, cholesterol, and blood sugar levels.

If you have already been diagnosed with CVD, there are a variety of treatments and management strategies that can help control the disease and reduce the risk of complications. These may include:

Medications: There are several types of medications that can be used to treat CVD, including blood pressure medications, cholesterol-lowering medications, and medications to prevent blood clots.

Medical procedures: Depending on the specific type of CVD, you may need to undergo a medical procedure such as angioplasty, stenting, or bypass surgery to improve blood flow to the heart or to prevent a stroke.

Lifestyle changes: Making healthy lifestyle changes, such as eating a healthy diet, getting regular physical activity, and quitting smoking, can help manage CVD and reduce the risk of complications.

Stress management: Managing stress through techniques such as meditation, yoga, or deep breathing can help reduce the risk of CVD complications.

By taking steps to prevent and manage CVD, you can significantly reduce your risk of developing serious complications and improve your overall quality of life.

Lifestyle Factors that Affect Cardiovascular Health
There are several lifestyle factors that can impact cardiovascular health and increase the risk of developing cardiovascular disease (CVD). These include:

Diet: A diet high in saturated and trans fats, salt, and added sugars can contribute to the development of CVD. On the other hand, a diet that is rich in fruits, vegetables, whole grains, and lean proteins can help reduce the risk of CVD.

Physical activity: Regular physical activity can help lower the risk of CVD by maintaining a healthy weight, controlling blood pressure, and improving cholesterol levels. Aim for at least 150 minutes of moderate-intensity exercise per week.

Smoking: Smoking damages the blood vessels and increases the risk of CVD.

Quitting smoking can significantly reduce the risk of CVD.

Alcohol consumption: Moderate alcohol consumption (up to one drink per day for women and two drinks per day for men) may have some protective effects on CVD, but excessive alcohol consumption can increase the risk of CVD.

Stress: Chronic stress can contribute to the development of CVD by increasing blood pressure and heart rate. Managing stress through techniques such as meditation, yoga, or deep breathing can help reduce the risk of CVD.

Sleep: Poor sleep quality and insufficient sleep have been linked to an increased risk of CVD. Aim for 7-9 hours of sleep per night.

By adopting a healthy lifestyle and managing these factors, you can significantly reduce your risk of developing CVD and improve your overall cardiovascular health.

Medical Treatment for Cardiovascular Disease

There are several types of medical treatments that can be used to manage cardiovascular disease (CVD) and reduce the risk of complications. These treatments may include

Medications: Depending on the specific type of CVD, you may be prescribed medications to help control the disease. These may include:

Blood pressure medications: These medications help lower blood pressure and reduce the strain on the heart and blood vessels. Examples include beta blockers, ACE inhibitors, and calcium channel blockers.

Cholesterol-lowering medications: These medications help lower levels of LDL cholesterol (the "bad" cholesterol) and reduce the risk of plaque buildup in the arteries. Examples include statins, fibrates, and bile acid sequestrants.

Blood thinners: These medications help prevent blood clots, which can cause a stroke or heart attack. Examples include aspirin, warfarin, and dabigatran.

Medical procedures: Depending on the specific type of CVD, you may need to undergo a medical procedure to improve blood flow to the heart or to prevent a stroke. These procedures may include:

Angioplasty: This procedure involves inserting a small balloon into the affected artery and inflating it to widen the artery and improve blood flow.

Stenting: This procedure involves inserting a small mesh tube (stent) into the affected artery to keep it open and improve blood flow.

Bypass surgery: This procedure involves creating a new path for blood to flow around a blocked artery, using a blood vessel from another part of the body.

Lifestyle changes: Making healthy lifestyle changes, such as eating a healthy diet, getting regular physical activity, and quitting smoking, can help manage CVD and reduce the risk of complications.

Stress management: Managing stress through techniques such as meditation, yoga, or deep breathing can help reduce the risk of CVD complications.

By working with your healthcare team and following your treatment plan, you can effectively manage CVD and reduce the risk of serious complications. It is important to take all medications as prescribed and to follow up with your healthcare provider regularly to monitor your condition and make any necessary adjustments to your treatment plan.

While medication and medical procedures may be necessary to manage cardiovascular disease (CVD), there are also a number of natural treatments that may be helpful in reducing the risk of CVD and improving overall cardiovascular health. These treatments may include:

Diet and nutrition: Adopting a healthy diet that is rich in fruits, vegetables, whole grains, and lean proteins can help reduce the risk of CVD. This may include following a Mediterranean diet, which is high in plant-based foods, healthy fats (such as olive oil), and seafood, and low in processed and red meats.

Physical activity: Regular physical activity can help lower the risk of CVD by maintaining a healthy weight, controlling blood pressure, and improving cholesterol levels. Aim for at least 150 minutes of moderate-intensity exercise per week.

Herbal remedies: Certain herbs and supplements may have potential benefits for CVD. However, it is important to speak with a healthcare provider before starting any new supplement, as some herbs can interact with medications or have potential side effects. Examples of herbs that may be helpful for CVD include garlic, hawthorn, and omega-3 fatty acids.

Stress management: Chronic stress can contribute to the development of CVD by increasing blood pressure and heart rate. Managing stress through techniques such as meditation, yoga, or deep breathing can help reduce the risk of CVD.

Sleep: Poor sleep quality and insufficient sleep have been linked to an increased risk of CVD. Aim for 7-9 hours of sleep per night and practice good sleep hygiene, such as avoiding screens before bed and creating a comfortable sleep environment.

It is important to remember that while natural treatments may be helpful in managing CVD, they should not be used as a replacement for medication or medical procedures. It is always best to work with a healthcare provider to determine the best treatment plan for your specific condition.

Alternative Therapies for Cardiovascular Disease

Alternative therapies are non-traditional approaches to healthcare that are not typically used in mainstream medicine. Some people with cardiovascular disease (CVD) may choose to use alternative therapies in addition to or instead of traditional medical treatments. However, it is important to keep in mind that the effectiveness of alternative therapies for CVD has not been extensively researched and they may not be as safe or effective as traditional medical treatments.

Some examples of alternative therapies that may be used for CVD include:

Acupuncture: Acupuncture is a form of traditional Chinese medicine that involves the insertion of thin needles into specific points on the body to stimulate the flow of energy. Some people with CVD may use acupuncture to help manage their condition, although the evidence for its effectiveness is mixed.

Chiropractic care: Chiropractic care involves the use of spinal manipulation to treat a variety of conditions, including CVD. While some people may find chiropractic care helpful for managing CVD, the evidence for its effectiveness is limited.

Herbal remedies: Certain herbs and supplements may have potential benefits for CVD. However, it is important to speak with a healthcare provider before starting any new supplement, as some herbs can interact with medications or have potential side effects. Examples of herbs that may be helpful for CVD include garlic, hawthorn, and omega-3 fatty acids.

Homeopathy: Homeopathy is a system of medicine that involves the use of highly diluted substances to stimulate the body's natural healing processes. Some people with CVD may use homeopathy to help manage their condition, although the evidence for its effectiveness is limited.

It is important to remember that alternative therapies should not be used as a replacement for traditional medical treatments for CVD. It is always best to work with a healthcare provider to determine the best treatment plan for your specific condition.

Conclusion

Cardiovascular disease (CVD) is a serious and potentially life-threatening condition that affects the heart and blood vessels. While there is no cure for CVD, it is a preventable and manageable disease through lifestyle changes, medication, and medical procedures.

Dr. Gregory K Edward's book on the prevention and management of CVD provides valuable advice for reducing the risk of CVD and effectively managing the condition. The book covers important topics such as identifying and addressing risk factors, adopting a healthy lifestyle, and utilizing medical treatments and alternative therapies to manage CVD.

Overall, Dr. Edward's book is an excellent resource for anyone looking to learn more about preventing and managing CVD. By following the advice in the book, you can significantly reduce your risk of developing serious complications and improve your overall quality of life.

cardiovascular disease (CVD) is a group of conditions that affect the heart and blood vessels, including coronary artery disease, heart failure, stroke, and hypertension. CVD is a leading cause of death and disability worldwide, but it is also preventable and manageable through lifestyle changes, medication, and medical procedures.

To prevent CVD, it is important to address risk factors such as high blood pressure, high cholesterol, diabetes, obesity, smoking, lack of physical activity, and poor diet. Adopting a healthy lifestyle that includes a healthy diet, regular physical activity, and stress management can significantly reduce the risk of CVD.

If you have already been diagnosed with CVD, there are a variety of treatments and management strategies that can help control the disease and reduce the risk of complications. These may include medications, medical procedures, lifestyle changes, and stress management.

By taking steps to prevent and manage CVD, you can significantly improve your cardiovascular health and reduce the risk of serious complications. It is important to work closely with your healthcare team to determine the best treatment plan for your specific condition.

The Importance of Maintaining a Healthy Cardiovascular System

The cardiovascular system is a complex network of the heart, blood vessels, and blood that plays a vital role in maintaining the overall health of the body. Maintaining a healthy cardiovascular system is important for a number of reasons, including:

Delivering oxygen and nutrients to the body: The cardiovascular system is responsible for transporting oxygen and nutrients from the lungs and digestive system to the cells and tissues throughout the body. This is essential for maintaining the proper function of the body's systems and organs.

Removing waste and toxins: The cardiovascular system also plays a role in the removal of waste and toxins from the body. The blood carries waste products and carbon dioxide away from the cells and to the liver and kidneys, where they are eliminated from the body.

Maintaining proper blood pressure: The cardiovascular system helps regulate blood pressure, which is the force of blood against the walls of the blood vessels. Maintaining normal blood pressure is important for proper organ function and to reduce the risk of CVD.

Supporting the immune system: The cardiovascular system is also involved in supporting the immune system, which helps protect the body from infections and diseases. The blood carries white blood cells and antibodies throughout the body to help fight off infections.

Facilitating physical activity: The cardiovascular system is essential for physical activity, as it helps deliver oxygen and nutrients to the muscles and remove waste products during exercise. Regular physical activity is important for maintaining a healthy cardiovascular system.

By maintaining a healthy cardiovascular system, you can improve your overall health and reduce the risk of CVD and other serious health problems. This can be achieved through a healthy diet, regular physical activity, and other lifestyle factors that support cardiovascular health. It is important to work with a healthcare provider to determine the best approach for maintaining a healthy cardiovascular system.

Steps to Take for Cardiovascular Disease Prevention and Management

Cardiovascular disease (CVD) is a group of conditions that affect the heart and blood vessels, including coronary artery disease, heart failure, stroke, and hypertension. CVD is a leading cause of death and disability worldwide, but it is also preventable and manageable through lifestyle changes and medical interventions. Here are some steps you can take to prevent and manage CVD:

Know your risk factors: CVD risk factors include high blood pressure, high cholesterol, diabetes, obesity, smoking, lack of physical activity, and poor diet. It is important to identify your risk factors and take steps to address them.

Adopt a healthy lifestyle: A healthy lifestyle can significantly reduce the risk of CVD. This includes eating a healthy diet that is rich in fruits, vegetables, whole grains, and lean proteins, getting regular physical activity, and not smoking or using tobacco products.

Manage stress: Chronic stress can contribute to the development of CVD. It is important to find ways to manage stress, such as through meditation, yoga, or deep breathing.

Get regular check-ups: Regular check-ups and screenings can help monitor your blood pressure, cholesterol, and blood sugar levels and allow for early identification and treatment of any potential issues.

Take medications as prescribed: If you have been prescribed medications to manage CVD, it is important to take them as directed. This includes taking them at the correct time and dosage and following any other instructions provided by your healthcare provider.

Follow your treatment plan: It is important to follow your treatment plan as prescribed by your healthcare provider. This may include making lifestyle changes, taking medications, and undergoing medical procedures as needed.

By following these steps, you can significantly reduce your risk of developing serious complications from CVD and improve your overall quality of life. It is important to work closely with your healthcare team to determine the best approach for preventing and managing CVD.

www.ingramcontent.com/pod-product-compliance
Lightning Source LLC
Chambersburg PA
CBHW070239220526
45465CB00004B/1451